6 Simple Rules
of Power

Discover how you can apply 6 simple habits that will **<u>change your life forever!</u>**

Terms and Conditions

LEGAL NOTICE

This book is not intended for use as a source of legal, business, accounting or financial advice. All readers are advised to seek services of competent professionals in legal, business, accounting and finance fields.

You are encouraged to print this book for easy reading.

Table Of Contents

Foreword

There's one thing that differentiates happy and successful individuals from misfortunate, unsuccessful individuals. It's all in the attitude and personal power.

We can't all of the time control the conditions that we chance upon, however what we may control is how we respond to them.

In that way we may make fresh selections and take a different action, therefore bringing ourselves toward success.

A positive mental attitude for life success is utterly crucial and provides great personal power.

Once you have an extremely positive attitude, you'll have a greater expectation of success and more personal power.

It forever appears that we get what we anticipate, and when you anticipate success and power that is precisely what you'll wind up discovering.

To help you formulate the sort of mental attitude that will bring success and personal power, I wish to share this book with you to help you accomplish better results.

6 Simple Rules Of Power

Discover how you can apply 6 simple habits that will change your life forever!

Chapter 1:
Successful Mental Picture

Synopsis

Forge and emboss indelibly on your brain a picture of yourself as succeeding. Hold this image doggedly. Never let it disappear. Your mind will look to formulate this image. Never consider yourself as bombing; never question the reality of the image. That's most serious, for the mind forever attempts to complete what it envisions. So forever picture "success" regardless how badly matters seem to be going at the present moment.

See It

To formulate your personal lucidity or purpose you have to do 3 things. 1st, define what success entails for you. 2nd, produce an intense mental image of you as a winner. 3rd, clear up your personal values. When you define what success entails for you personally, I advise that you formulate a well-defined mental picture of you as a success. This picture ought to be as graphic as you are able to you make it.

When I was twenty, I called forth a picture of myself as a successful speaker, personal coach, business consultant and writer. I worked from my home base -- where I composed and formulated the programs I pitched at customer locations. This office had a floor to ceiling wall of books that I may utilize for easy reference. It likewise had a typewriter and a huge, clunky phone. Personal computers and the net were not around in the early 70's.

I likewise viewed myself having one to one discussions with senior leadership in an assortment of organizations, carrying on education and team building sittings in conference rooms at their businesses. Astonishingly, a lot of the individuals in the sessions were having cigarettes. I had really graphic images of standing before big audiences at sales meetings performing talks. I visualized myself signing a book I had composed at a bookshop. I likewise viewed myself on planes, traveling to my speech production, training and consulting gigs.

All of these graphic pictures came true. My office is very much like I had envisaged it -- except it has a 2 personal computers and a cell, not a typewriter and clumsy telephone set. The hordes of books are there

-- brimming over. I've composed 20 of the books on the shelf. Individuals don't have cigarettes in my training and team building sittings any longer and I utilize slides rather than handwritten charts, but the big things are the same as I'd thought. I've talked to audiences all over the world. I've racked up many frequent flyer miles.

I'm living my aspiration -- in large part since I dared to aspire to it a long time ago. What's your aspiration? Can you produce a graphic mental image of it? I advise that you take a little time for yourself. Ask and answer these 3 things:

Where do I wish to be ten, twenty and thirty years from today? How will it look and feel when I get there? How will my life be?

Ask and resolve any additional questions that will help you formulate a clear-cut, intense mental image of your success. This isn't day dreaming. It's true work. You're contriving your future in your mind. Keep this impression with you as you set about your daily business.

Every once in a while, enquire of yourself if what you did that day got you any closer to your image of success. In that way, you'll be holding your dream alive -- and moving towards your destination.

The horse sense point here is easy. Successful individuals specify what success signifies to them. Then they formulate a compelling and clear-cut image of their success. They utilize this mental image to help hold their aspirations alive and to keep moving forward to what they wish in their lives and vocations. Producing an intense mental image of your success isn't day dreaming. It's true work -- the work of contriving your future, so you are able to take the steps essential to produce it.

Chapter 2:
Cancel The Negative

Synopsis

If a negative thought bearing on your personal power springs to mind, intentionally voice a positive thought to invalidate it.

Thoughts

Most individuals utilize affirmations, meditation, visual images or additional exercises to bump off negative thoughts so they may create fresh things in their life (that may be money, success, love, and so forth.).

Regrettably, with 95% of our thoughts being damaging, and most of these living in our subconscious mind, it may take a lot of years to produce alteration in our lives. You have to be able to discover the blocks that are holding you back so that you are able to produce the success you wish in your life.

It put up be really hard to shift your focus when it's something that's really crucial to you, or if the trouble seems overpowering.

Weight loss is a good example of this. When you feel plump, you can't get lean. How come? Well, while you feel plump, you tend to get blue or depressed, then you might consume more or you might sleep more to battle the blue feelings you're having. If you center on feeling plump (the trouble), chances are you'll draw in more of that to you and acquire even more weight.

On the other hand, if you center on the resolution (acquiring more physical exercise, eating sounder), you'll be prompted to take action and you'll draw in the support and tools you require to accomplish your goal.

So, by switching your focus from the trouble to the resolution, you will draw in what you wish into your life rather than what you don't want.

Chapter 3:
Deal With Difficulties

Synopsis

Don't develop obstacles in your imagination. Devaluate every alleged obstruction. Downplay them. Troubles must be examined and efficiently dealt with to be done away with, however they must be seen for only what they are. And therefore not be amplified by fear thoughts.

Problems

Troubles can't be avoided in day-to-day life. When we don't have troubles, the human mind has a propensity to produce additional issues. To deal with troubles that come up we shouldn't seek to quash them. We have to look at them as a chance to better our nature. By defeating problems we may beef up our will and learn useful lessons.

Here are a few hints for addressing troubles:

1. Do not feel misfortunate

The existence of an issue doesn't mean we ought to feel misfortunate or shamed. True, the trouble might be the consequence of our previous errors, but, regretting the past times won't help us deal with the subject at hand. In addition to that, rather often troubles come up through no fault of our own. To feel shamed for issues produced by other people is to make a double error.

2. A Chance not a trouble

A great deal of the time what we see as a trouble is truly a chance to learn something or get over a particular weakness. We'll never ask in issues into our life, but if we're able to have the correct mental attitude we recognize that by defeating them we may learn something rather useful.

3. Remain resolute

If the issue is stemming from others, we must be staunch in not allowing the issue to enter into us. We ought to attempt to build up an invisible roadblock to stop the negativity getting into us. For instance, if other people are very strained, they'll subconsciously try to pass their anxieties onto us. If we're not solid these anxieties will move into us. All the same, if we may detach ourselves from their concerns and stress we'll stay untouched.

4. Envisage the resolution.

If we simply center on the issues facing us, we'll become dejected and our focus will be on the magnitude of the trouble. In that frame of mind it gets to be an uphill battle to work out the issue. To subdue a problem we have to center on the resolution. Consequently, we have to retain a positive mental attitude and take pragmatic steps to figure out a solution, bit-by-bit.

5. Alter our mental attitude

Rather often particular issues keep duplicating themselves. These troubles are the result of our inside and outer mental attitude. For these recurrent issues we have to produce a fresh view. It's insufficient to attempt and prevent these issues or react with our habitual response. If advantageous take the advice of others. This will help you to step back and view the issue from another angle. The crucial thing is to alter our mind-set. Issues only go away when we subdue the problem at the root. The root cause is our idea and position.

6. Use humor

Humor may be an effective counter poison to a lot of issues of the mind. If we have little concerns and headaches attempt to smile and laugh. – It might just be the most beneficial answer.

Chapter 4:
Be Yourself

Synopsis

Don't be in awe of others and try to imitate them. Nobody may be you as efficiently as you are able to. Remember likewise that most individuals, in spite of their confident appearance and behavior, are a great deal of the time as scared as you are and as in question of themselves.

Be You

Being yourself is observing you, as an individual - finding out how to express yourself and be pleased with who you are. For a few individuals, it's finding out how to love yourself, for other people, it's not shrouding who you are or altering things about you to fit in.

Specify yourself. You can't be yourself if you don't understand, know, and live with yourself first. It ought to be your basic goal to discover this. Attempt to take time for yourself and chew over your life and selections. Attempt to consider what sort of things you would or wouldn't like to accomplish, and behave accordingly; discovering through trial and error helps more than you may believe it does. You are able to even take personality quizzes, but be heedful to only take what you wish from them and not let them specify you.

Work at accepting errors and selections you've arrived at; they're complete and in the past, so there's no use howling over spilled milk. Quit caring about how individuals perceive you. The truth is, it truly doesn't matter. It's unimaginable to be yourself when you're caught up in questioning "Do they think I'm comical? Does she think I'm plump? Do they believe I'm unintelligent?" To be yourself, you've got to release these concerns and just let your conduct flow, with only your thoughtfulness of other people as a filter — not their consideration of you.

Besides, if you alter yourself for one person or group, a different individual or group might not like you, and you may go around in a vicious circle trying to please individuals; it's altogether pointless in the long run, and it leaves you depleted. All the same, if somebody you trust and regard critiques facets of who you are, feel free to gauge (truthfully) whether or not it's precise rather than living with or dismissing the critique categorically.

Be truthful and open. What have you got to conceal? We're all fallible, growing, learning humans. If you feel ashamed or speculative about any facet of yourself — and you sense that you have to shroud those parts of you, whether physically or emotionally — then you have to come to terms with that and learn to change over your alleged defects into individualistic oddities. Be truthful with yourself, but don't bash yourself; utilize this doctrine with other people, likewise.

There's a difference between being decisive and being truthful; learn to watch the manner in which you say things to yourself and other people when being truthful.

Loosen up. Quit worrying about the worst that may occur, particularly in social spots. So what if you founder? Or get food in your teeth?

Discover how to laugh at yourself both when it occurs and later on. Turn it into a good story that you are able to share with other people. It lets them understand that you're not perfect and makes you feel more relaxed, also. It's likewise a magnetic quality for somebody to be able to laugh at

themselves and not take themselves too
earnestly!

Acquire and express your individualism. Whether it's your feel of style, or even your style of talking, if your favored way of doing something wanders from the mainstream, then be pleased with it... unless it's destructive to yourself or other people. Have a rich day. Trust in who you are. If you're forever working to be somebody you're not, you'll never be a pleased individual. Be yourself and demonstrate to the world you're pleased with the way you are! Nobody understands you better than you and that's how it ought to be.

You deserve to be your own best admirer, so begin trying to work out how you are able to do that. If you had to be with yourself for a day, what is the most amusing sort of individual you could be, while still representing yourself? What is the most beneficial version of you?

Trust in this theme and utilize that as your beginning point.

Love and live with yourself as you are today. Abide by your own flair. The basic thing a lot of individuals do is copy other's actions as it appears like the more beneficial route to fit in, but truly, shouldn't you stick out? Sticking out is really difficult, yes, but you want to try to avoid donning other people's views of you.

Even if it's not something you'd commonly do; that's what representing yourself is all about. Perhaps you like to sit outdoors on the deck under an umbrella in the midst of the rain, perhaps you've different ideas of matters, instead of others, perhaps you like strawberry cake rather than the basic chocolate cake, whatever you are, admit it. Being dissimilar is utterly beautiful and it draws individuals to you....

Chapter 5:
Get Counseling

Synopsis

Acquire a competent counselor to help you comprehend why you do what you do. Learn of the beginning of your inferiority and self-distrust feelings which frequently start out in childhood. Self-cognition leads to a remedy.......

Seek Help

Ask yourself a few questions:

➢ Are you seeking group or individual therapy? Couples therapy? Family therapy? Are you seeking short, solution-focused therapy or long-run, in-depth work?

➢ What issues do you wish to work at? What do you desire to achieve? Do you have a taste as to what therapeutic mode (like verbal therapy, art, movement...) you wish to work in?

➢ Do you favor a male or female therapist? Does it make whatever difference to you?

➢   Are you available during the day or do you require evening/weekend sittings? What locations are handy for you?

➢   What fee can you give? Do you require a sliding scale?

Arrive at a list of potential therapists and their numbers:

Talk to acquaintances, loved ones and other people who might be able to refer you to a therapist. Other references for discovering a therapist are ads, referral services, and local schools and the net.

Get hold of the therapist you wish to understand more about. Let them know you're shopping around.

A few therapists will speak with you on the telephone and you are able to acquire a sense of them and their work. Other people want to talk on the telephone briefly and then start regular sittings. Still other people offer one session at no charge.

Whatever the therapist's initial policy, you are able to help yourself get a great match. You've the right to ask questions. A few questions you may ask are:

- ➤ What is your preparation?
- ➤ How long have you been in practice?
- ➤ How much do you charge?
- ➤ When do you visit clients?
- ➤ How soon may I acquire an appointment?
- ➤ Have you ever been in therapy?
- ➤ What troubles do you work with?
- ➤ What do you specialize in?

> What experience do you have with the trouble that I wish to work on? Can you assist me? If not, will you refer me to a different therapist?

> How would we work together on subjects?

> How long will it call for?

As you arrive at your conclusion, believe your gut instinct! No sum of training, paperwork or government ordinance may ever substitute for your own personal feel of what is most beneficial for you.

Do any of these therapists appear to be correct for you?

Do you feel safe with him/her? Do you feel you may connect with and work with this therapist? Is he/she easy with you and your issues?

As you go along in therapy, speak to your therapist about your advancement. You've a right to ask questions and to get replies to them.

You, the client, are forever in charge of your operation. You've the right to turn down what your therapist is providing you. You've the right to change therapists and/or styles of therapy.

Intimate conduct and/or contact between therapist and client are NEVER accepted behavior.

Outside relationships like business, friendly relationship and socializing with your therapist are likewise not acceptable as they produce roadblocks to the therapeutic procedure.

Do you sense that you're relating with your therapist? Feelings of uncomfortableness are to be anticipated in therapy, however feeling unsafe with your therapist is a major cautionary sign to you.

Chapter 6:

Develop Self Respect

Synopsis

Make a truthful approximation of your own power, and then raise it 10%. Don't get narcissistic, but acquire a wholesome self-regard. Trust in your own god issued powers.

Self Regard

Self-regard is key for a dandy life. If we lack self-respect, we'll be insecure and endeavor to be person we're not. To develop self-regard means to cultivate the self-assurance to manage whatever life casts at us. The following are a few ways we may better our self-regard.

Remember, self-regard comes from an inner belief and not an egoistic feeling of superiority.

1. Be truthful to yourself

There's great social pressing from parents, work and society to become a particular individual and to accomplish particular things. It's a pressing difficult to detach from. But a true self-regard only comes from being truthful to our inner calling. It's crucial you've faith in your own values and remember what is significant to you. Just because others believe you ought to act in a particular way, doesn't mean they're correct. Everybody needs to abide by their own path.

Even if other people don't honor your decision, it's crucial that you do. Simply ask yourself whether you come into the world to delight Tom, Dick and Harry or inhabit your own life?

2. Discover how to manage critique

We're tender beings. Nobody wishes criticism and when we're picked apart, either forthwith or indirectly, we feel badly about ourself – even if the critique isn't warranted. To sustain a sense of self-regard, we have to learn how to manage criticism. Don't take critique personally. View it from a separated perspective. Perhaps it's untrue, in which case we ought to ignore it. If their is a little truth, we may utilize it to grow our character. But, it's crucial not to take critique too personally. Just because we're not really good at a specific task, doesn't mean we have to lose our self-regard.

3. Look nice without being a slave to style

Our visual aspect is crucial. It may provide us confidence or it may make us feel clumsy. Take care of your visual aspect; dressing smart for the correct occasion gives us self-assurance. At the same time, we don't wish to be the slave of style trends. Dress for your own advantage; don't dress in the anticipation of pleasing other people and getting complements.

4. Prevent green-eyed monster

Jealousy of others success is a basic way of losing our happiness and self-regard. Jealousy is merely envy of others success. We feel misfortunate that we can't enjoy their success. Occasionally it may even lead us to criticizing the other individual. If we abide by this path of jealousy we'll decidedly lose our sense of self-regard. When we're constantly equating ourselves to others, we're stating our self-regard depends on being better than other people. But, the fact is, there will always be a few individuals more successful than ourself. The trick to persistent self-regard is to be happy through others success. We ought to never feel that others success in any way decreases our self worth.

5. Respect other people

If you've no regard for other people, how can you have self-regard? Self-regard means we have an inner assurance and inner confidence, but this isn't a confidence built upon superiority. It's the wrong approach to attempt and feel better by putting other people down. If we seek the good qualities in others, it's easier to remember the great qualities in ourselves.

6. Never detest yourself

We make errors, we might do the improper thing; but we ought to never put ourselves down unnecessarily. If we're not heedful we begin bitterly regretting matters and even disliking ourselves. We ought to never detest our self, it's very destructive. Listen to your moral sense, but, don't be too hard on yourself and feel loaded down with guilt.

7. Forgive

Forgive other people and forgive yourself. Don't live in the past tense, but, go on from past errors and hard situations. If your mind is absorbed with issues from the past, you'll forever feel guilty and despicable. Don't let your self worth be determined by past errors.

8. Be selfless

The way to self-regard isn't through a distended sense of pride; this is a fake type of self-regard. We might think that the praise of others supercharges our self-regard, but, really this praise brings on a vulnerable ego. If our self-regard is based on the praise of other people then our self-regard will be very flimsy. Self-regard shouldn't be contingent on the praise of others; it ought to be independent of others praise.

Wrapping Up

Keep going following up on your goals, desires, and ambitions with ambition, trust, and a positive mental attitude.

Outfitted with these traits, nobody can fail. A positive attitude for success will conquer all and provide you great personal power.